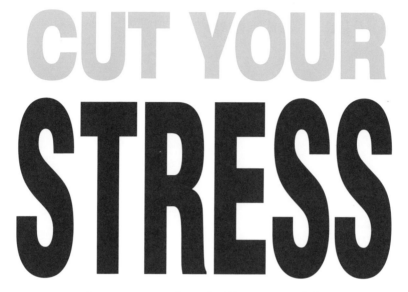

CUT YOUR
STRESS

An easy-to-follow guide to stress-free living

Quercus

CONTENTS

WHAT IS STRESS?

Stress is a modern term, used to describe the unpleasant physical and emotional symptoms people experience when under excess pressure.

A certain amount of pressure is beneficial – it gets you out of bed in the mornings and primes you to meet life's challenges. Stress develops only when the pressure rises above the level at which you feel able to cope. This level varies from person to person, and also from time to time, as it depends on many factors.

WHEN STRESSED, YOU MAY DESCRIBE YOURSELF AS:

- Shattered
- Drained
- Anxious
- Tense
- On edge
- Hassled
- Uptight
- About to explode
- At the end of your tether
- Desperate for a drink or smoke

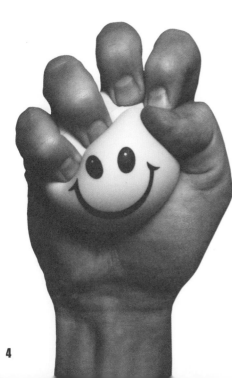

When you are fit, well fed, have had a refreshing night's sleep, are in a rewarding relationship and have money in the bank, you can handle more pressure than when you are unfit, skip meals, lack sleep and are overdrawn – especially if you've also just had a row with your partner.

Feeling stressed simply means you are under more pressure (real or imagined) than you feel comfortable with at a certain point. You start to feel uneasy, your mouth goes dry, your hands feel clammy and your legs turn to jelly. You may develop a lump in your throat and a characteristic sinking feeling in the pit of your stomach.

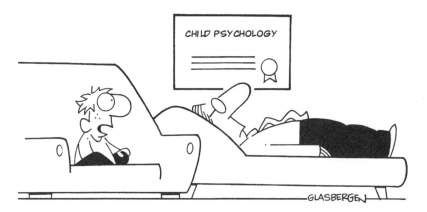

'You're spending the best years of your life doing a job
that you hate so that you can buy stuff you don't need to
support a lifestyle you don't enjoy. Sounds crazy to me!'

STRESSORS Events or situations that provoke stress are known as stressors. Some will cause most people to become stressed whenever they occur. Good examples are environmental changes that overstimulate the senses, including excessive noise, blinding light, extremes of temperature and overcrowding.

Other situations, such as public speaking, are stressful for many but not all people. An experienced presenter will approach an after-dinner speech, for example, in a relaxed frame of mind – especially if the person thrives on being the centre of attention. This is because familiarity with a situation, along with your personality type, influences how you respond to potential stressors.

Conversely, lack of pressure can also lead to stress if you are stuck in a rut and feel frustrated by too little stimulation or satisfaction.

COPING WITH STRESS The subjective nature of stress means that it's possible to change the way you respond to stress, so that you deal with things more calmly and constructively. And, once you identify the stressors in your life, you can make plans to overcome them successfully.

The approaches outlined in this book will help you to raise the bar on your comfort zone, with the result that your perception of how much stress you can deal with is increased.

THE 'FIGHT-OR-FLIGHT' RESPONSE

The symptoms of stress are produced by your body's
'fight-or-flight' response, which is driven by hormones
from your adrenal glands.

When confronted with a potential danger that may require physical exertion (that is, fighting or fleeing), your nervous system triggers the release of stress hormones from the adrenal glands. Within seconds of spotting a hungry tiger running at you, the levels of adrenaline/epinephrine in your blood rise as much as 1,000-fold. This produces a noticeable jolt as your systems go onto 'red alert'.

FIGHT ...

BLOOD GLUCOSE LEVELS
RISE TO PROVIDE INSTANT
ENERGY ... YOUR MUSCLES
ARE NOW PRIMED FOR
EXTRA POWER

CIRCULATION Your heart pumps faster, and your pulse races. As your heart contracts with increased force, your blood pressure rises to send more oxygen-rich blood to your muscles and brain. Blood diverts away from your intestines towards your brain and muscles. Your blood also becomes more 'sticky', to limit bleeding should injury occur.

THE ADRENAL GLANDS

You have two adrenal (also sometimes called suprarenal) glands, one above each kidney. These small, triangular structures have an outer cortex, which produces the stress hormone cortisol, and an inner medulla that generates the stress hormones adrenaline (or epinephrine), noradrenaline (or norepinephrine) and dopamine.

RESPIRATION Your airways widen and your breathing rate increases. This typically starts with a sudden intake of breath – the gasp of fear – which allows more oxygen to flood into your lungs.

MUSCLES Your muscles tense for action. You stiffen and tremble with fear, and your voice becomes high-pitched and shaky. Your blood glucose levels rise to provide instant energy. Your muscles are now primed for extra power and speed – often leading to extraordinary feats of strength.

NERVOUS SYSTEM Increased blood flow to your brain improves your memory and your ability to think straight. This helps you to plan your way out of a tricky situation. Your pupils dilate and your eyes widen with fear, enabling you to spot danger from farther afield. Your sensory perception becomes more acute, especially your hearing, while your sensitivity to pain reduces. Injuries often go unnoticed until you reach a place of safety.

INTERNAL ORGANS Your bowels, bladder and stomach empty to make you lighter for running. You may wet yourself, experience nervous diarrhoea or even vomit through fear. Circulation to the gut shuts down as blood diverts to your muscles, causing so-called 'butterflies' in your stomach.

In males, stress causes the testicles to be drawn up towards the abdomen, for safe keeping.

SKIN You may blanche with fear, as blood drains from your skin to your brain and muscles. This is followed by flushing as your sweat glands switch on, and blood diverts back to the surface, ready for rapid cooling after running or fighting. You literally go clammy with fear.

The symptoms of the fight-or-flight reaction mobilize energy within the body, priming you for vigorous physical exertion. If this energy is not consumed, the effects of stress continue to build up, draining the body of energy. One of the best ways to switch off the effects of stress and promote the more beneficial 'rest-and-digest' response is therefore through non-competitive exercise.

... OR FLIGHT
YOUR BOWELS, BLADDER AND STOMACH EMPTY ... TO MAKE YOU LIGHTER FOR RUNNING

CAUSES OF STRESS

Almost anything can lead to stress if it makes you feel angry, tense, frustrated or unhappy. Stress can result from work, finances, relationships, bereavement, your environment or your interaction with certain people.

The common underlying theme is often change. Too much change, too quickly, is highly stressful – especially when it is imposed on you without your consent. Change is produced by major life events such as marriage, starting a new job, winning the lottery, having a baby or experiencing a bereavement or serious illness. Sometimes it's easy to pinpoint a major life event as a cause of stress, but there may also be no obvious single cause. It can result from the buildup of a number of small things, which, added together, make the final straw that breaks the proverbial camel's back.

Look at the table opposite. The more of these life events you have experienced over the past year, particularly those rated as very high or high, the more likely you are to be experiencing significant stress.

INTERNAL VERSUS EXTERNAL CAUSES OF STRESS

Most life events are external causes of stress – they happen around you or are imposed upon you. There are also some important internal causes of stress. These include physical tiredness, mental exhaustion, hormone changes (for example, menstruation, menopause), lack of fitness, disrupted biorhythms and negative self-image and thoughts. If you think you aren't good enough, or that you won't be able to cope, then these become self-fulfilling prophecies. If you believe you ARE good enough, and are determined to cope, then you will keep trying until you succeed.

This is where personality plays a key role in determining how you respond to change, and whether you perceive that change as a desirable opportunity (positive pressure) or a dangerous threat (negative stress).

Severe anxiety that follows on from a traumatic event is known as post-traumatic stress disorder (PTSD).

Death of a partner
Divorce or separation
Going to jail
Death of a close relative
Personal injury or illness
Marriage

VERY HIGH

Loss of your job
Moving house
Getting back together with a partner after a separation
Retiring
Serious illness of a close relative
Pregnancy
Sexual difficulties
New baby
Changing your job
Financial problems
Death of close friend

HIGH

Family arguments
Having a large mortgage or loan
Legal action as a result of debts
Change in work responsibilities
Offspring leaving home
Trouble with in-laws
Outstanding personal achievement
Partner begins or stops work
Starting or finishing college
Change in living conditions
New Year's resolutions to change personal habits
Stopping smoking or drinking
Trouble with your boss at work

MODERATE

Change in your working hours or conditions
Change of residence
Change of school
Change in recreational activities
Change in social activities
Change in sleeping habits, eg due to shift work
Change in eating habits, eg to lose weight, lower cholesterol
Having a small mortgage or loan
Having a holiday (think of all those travel delays)
Christmas
Minor run-ins with the law

LOW

LIFE EVENT

STRESS LEVEL

*Adapted from Holmes & Rahe

PERSONALITY TYPES You are an individual, and your unique personality plays a large part in how you cope with stress.

The latest research suggests that your personality type can be defined according to five factors. These are your:

1 openness to new experiences (likelihood of being adventurous, curious)
2 conscientiousness (tendency to be self-disciplined, purposeful and persistent)
3 extraversion and introversion (willingness to be the centre of attention and meet new people)
4 agreeableness (predisposition to be easygoing, cooperative and compassionate)
5 neuroticism, or emotional instability (readiness to experience negative emotions, such as anger, anxiety, irritation and frustration).

You score somewhere on the scale from high to low for each of these five factors. The resulting overall blend determines whether you perceive change as positive pressure, or as negative stress.

If you are very open to new experiences, you will cope better with change, and experience less stress as a result, than someone who is less adventurous.

If you are very conscientious, you will experience more stress when change disrupts your schedules and you don't get things done than someone who is less conscientious.

If you are extroverted and approach new situations enthusiastically, and with a positive frame of mind, you will find changing situations and meeting new people less stressful than someone who is more introverted.

If you are a highly agreeable person, you are more likely to let change wash over you then someone who is disagreeable and less willing to put themselves out.

And, finally, if you score highly in terms of neuroticism, you are more vulnerable to stress than those who are more emotionally stable – you are more likely to interpret situations as threatening or difficult.

How you respond to stress is not set in stone, however. The good news is that by learning how to recognize any unhelpful thought patterns and behaviours that increase your experience of stress, you can replace them with strategies that will help you to cope more effectively.

Realign your priorities and aim for what's worth being, rather than what's worth having. Try to gain a sense of what the present moment is about.

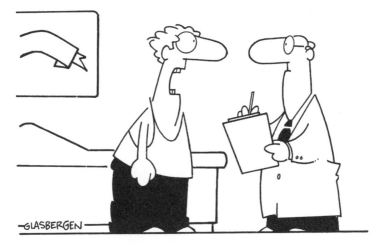

'I'm learning how to relax, doctor –
but I want to relax *better* and *faster!*
I want to be on the cutting edge of relaxation!'

STRESS ADDICTS

Some people are so used to feeling stressed that a highly strung state seems normal and they find it hard to relax.

They are addicted to the buzz-like adrenaline high associated with stress. These people, who like to live in the fast lane and who need a lot of sensation and stimulation, score highly on the extraversion scale.

You may be addicted to stress if you:
- feel high after successfully finishing a demanding, stressful task
- deliberately pile on the pressure, scheduling more and more into less and less time
- always play to win
- choose to work long hours at the expense of social and family life
- find it difficult to sit down, relax and do nothing
- become angry, aggressive and impatient with delays, queues or lack of punctuality in others.

People who are addicted to stress will experience burn-out sooner or later, experiencing stress-related symptoms such as insomnia, headache, poor concentration, irritability and reduced performance. If they don't slow down, and learn how to cope with their stress, they are heading for health problems such as high blood pressure and a heart attack or stroke.

WHY STRESS IS HARMFUL

When the pressure you're under exceeds your ability to cope, it has an adverse effect on your health. It can worsen conditions such as eczema and irritable bowel syndrome, and contribute to high blood pressure, coronary artery disease and stroke. Stress reduces immunity, so you are more prone to infections. It may also raise your risk of cancer. In addition, it makes you more likely to rely on emotional crutches such as alcohol, nicotine and recreational drugs.

PANIC ATTACKS

When you experience stress, your breathing rate increases as part of the fight-or-flight response. As well as drawing more oxygen into your lungs, you breath out more carbon dioxide (CO_2), an acidic waste gas. This is fine when you are generating more CO_2 through strenuous exercise. When you are stressed at a desk, however, exhaling too much carbon dioxide makes your blood increasingly alkaline. This affects your nerve function to produce physical symptoms such as dizziness, faintness, pins and needles, ringing in the ears and anxiety. It can also lead to a panic attack.

If you feel panic rising, consciously slow your breathing and, if necessary, breathe in and out of your cupped hands. This is less conspicuous than breathing through the traditional paper bag.

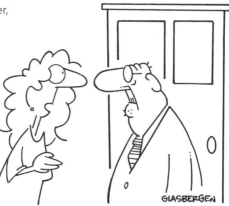

GLASBERGEN

'Honey, when you left for the office this morning, you were a happy, enthusiastic, vibrant 25-year-old! Do you want to talk about it?'

stress → messages to brain → shallow rapid breathing → exhaling excess CO_2 → alkaline blood → increased anxiety and panic → stress

ANXIETY CYCLE Long-term stress can trigger a cycle of anxiety as shown, right. People who habitually hyperventilate (overbreathe) experience a frightening number of physical symptoms, including difficulty breathing, a lump in the throat, chest pain, palpitations, visual disturbances, numbness, severe headache, insomnia and even collapse.

Caution: It is important to seek medical advice if these symptoms occur – don't diagnose a panic attack yourself, or a more serious problem may be missed.

PHOBIAS Long-term stress can lead to complex social phobias that are grounded in negative thoughts, such as worrying about not being able to cope or having nothing interesting to say, or being embarrassed in front of others.

Someone with a social anxiety disorder tends to think everyone is more competent in public than they are, and small things such as forgetting someone's name, blushing, having to introduce yourself to strangers, or just walking into a crowded room can become a major ordeal.

Another common fear is agoraphobia, which is often described as fear of open spaces. It is, however, more complicated, and includes the fear of unfamiliar or crowded places or even going out alone. The person may be confined to home through a fear of being judged by others.

PROLONGED STRESS CAN CONTRIBUTE TO:

- Reduced immunity
- Eczema
- Low sex drive
- Tension headaches
- Asthma
- Insomnia
- Poor glucose control
- High blood pressure
- Coronary artery disease
- Anxiety disorder
- Panic attacks
- Irritable bowel syndrome
- Tiredness all the time
- Psoriasis
- Erectile dysfunction
- Migraine
- Trichotillomania (pulling out body hair)
- Indigestion
- Peptic ulcers
- Increased risk of accident
- Type 2 diabetes
- Abnormal blood clotting
- Stroke
- Teeth grinding
- Depressive illness
- Cancer

RECOGNIZING YOUR STRESS SIGNALS

Doing something about stress is relatively easy – the difficult thing is acknowledging and accepting that you are experiencing excess pressure. Becoming familiar with the symptoms of stress means you can adapt to reduce the pressures in your life and cope more effectively. Tick any of the following traits that you recognize in yourself:

EARLY-WARNING SIGNS

Do you feel:
- ☐ uneasy
- ☐ on edge
- ☐ tense
- ☐ flustered
- ☐ uptight?

PSYCHOLOGICAL SYMPTOMS

Do you experience:
- ☐ frustration
- ☐ difficulty concentrating
- ☐ muddled thinking
- ☐ a tendency to lose perspective
- ☐ difficulty making rational decisions
- ☐ a tendency to make rash decisions
- ☐ negative thoughts
- ☐ loss of self-confidence
- ☐ lost sense of humour
- ☐ feelings of impending doom?

Onychophagia, better known as nail biting, is a common response to stress. Behavioural treatments aim to replace the habit with one that is less harmful, such as biting something else (for example, carrot sticks or chewing gum).

EMOTIONAL SYMPTOMS

Do you easily become or feel:
- ☐ irritable
- ☐ angry
- ☐ isolated
- ☐ defensive
- ☐ hopeless
- ☐ hostile
- ☐ guilty
- ☐ aggressive?

PHYSICAL SYMPTOMS

Do you regularly experience any of these symptoms:
- ☐ sweaty palms
- ☐ dry mouth
- ☐ rapid pulse
- ☐ tense muscles
- ☐ lump in the throat
- ☐ butterflies in your stomach
- ☐ trembling
- ☐ urinary frequency (habitual need to go to the toilet)
- ☐ nervous diarrhoea
- ☐ erratic breathing with a tendency to hyperventilate
- ☐ panic attacks?

If these physical effects of the fight-or-flight response are allowed to continue in the long term, your body will become drained of energy and you may develop the following:

- tiredness all the time
- insomnia
- tension headaches
- indigestion
- nausea
- loss of sex drive
- sexual difficulties.

BEHAVIOURAL SYMPTOMS

As you feel more and more stressed, you may develop behavioural strategies that, although they may make you feel better in the short term, affect your long-term health and further undermine your ability to cope.

You may become:

- reliant on alcohol
- reliant on cigarettes
- reliant on other recreational drugs.

In addition, you may:

- comfort eat
- skip meals
- display disordered eating behaviour, such as anorexia nervosa or bulimia
- become socially withdrawn
- develop obsessive or compulsive behaviour.

By learning to recognize the symptoms of stress, you can step in to stop its increasingly harmful, downward spiral, which, ultimately, can lead to a nervous breakdown – total inability to cope with life.

GENERALIZED ANXIETY DISORDER (GAD) is diagnosed when someone has spent at least six months worrying excessively about a number of everyday problems. People with GAD are always anticipating disaster and are unable to relax because of worries about health, finances, family, career – or even just the thought of having to get through the day. Depression can also occur, with feelings of sadness, hopelessness, loss of appetite and early-morning waking.

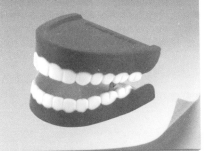

DO YOU GRIND YOUR TEETH WHEN STRESSED?

Known as bruxism, this can occur during sleep or while awake. You could be a grinder if your teeth look worn-down, flattened or chipped; if you develop increased tooth sensitivity; or if you wake with jaw pain, tightness in your jaw muscles, earache, a dull headache or have chewed tissue on the inside of your cheeks. Ask your bed partner if he or she ever hears you gnashing your teeth during the night.

KEEPING A STRESS DIARY
Filling in a stress diary for at least a week helps you to pinpoint your stressors. Keep your diary pages close by so you can make notes after each stressful event (see pages 54-55 for a blank template). This is a useful exercise that is worth repeating regularly.

Here's an example of a completed stress diary:

Date:	**Day:** Monday	Tuesday	Wednesday

Time of day	Intensity of stress (1-10)	Situation (causes, places, people)	How I felt
05.30	6	Awoke early due to noisy barking of neighbour's dog	Angry, annoyed, tired
08.40	5	Stuck in traffic jam on way to work	Frustrated, aggressive
10.40	8	Yelled at by boss over late delivery of stock and loss of sales; but it's out of my control	Defensive – it's not my fault; rapid pulse; felt trembly, tense and sick
18.00	6	Shopping for supper – long queue with only one very slow girl on the check-out	Frustrated; hungry; irritable
19.00	7	Yelled at partner for not helping to prepare supper	Unappreciated; put-upon; hostile

Record how you feel at the time. When you later recognize any negative responses that were triggered by the event, note these down, too. Having identified the problems, think about possible solutions. Consider how you might cope better with each stressor if it were to recur. Where appropriate, you might plan how to avoid some stressful situations altogether, such as shopping at busy times. Avoidance is not always appropriate,

however – you can't avoid someone who causes you stress at work, for example. These situations are best dealt with by changing how you respond to them. And remember, just because a situation is stressful now (such as public speaking), if you keep doing it, it will become familiar enough that you no longer perceive it as a threat. Successful people say 'Yes' to positive pressure; others get scared and say 'No' to the perceived threat.

Thursday	Friday	Saturday	Sunday

Negative responses (including rises in blood pressure)	**Possible solutions**
Yelled at family members; threw shoe out of the window in direction of dog	Speak to neighbours; wear a sleep mask designed to reduce light and sound; consider moving (more stress!); buy new shoes
Drove erratically; jumped a traffic light	Leave home earlier on Tuesdays, which are always busy because of market; listen to calming music or a talking book
Was tearful; he's an idiot; ate a doughnut with my coffee, even though I'm trying to lose weight; blood pressure raised	Negotiate reduced costs for breach of contract with current supplier; research alternative suppliers and discuss solutions with the boss (who's obviously stressed out, too); avoid staff canteen – take water and fruit to work instead
Snapped at girl; forgot to buy bread	Order shopping online for home delivery
Had a stiff gin and tonic, followed by half a bottle of wine; blood pressure raised	Go for run after work to burn off stresses of the day; cut back on alcohol – try a relaxing herbal tea instead

MEDICAL APPROACHES

At one time, the medical treatment of stress involved the use of tranquillizers such as benzodiazepine drugs. These anti-anxiety pills did not address the causes of stress, but numbed the person's response so they no longer felt the pressure.

Although this may seem a good idea, benzodiazepines have a high potential for addiction. They are now used only occasionally, for short periods of time, to treat acute stress. A doctor is more likely to offer a sick note, if the stress is work-related, or may suggest cognitive behaviour therapy (CBT) or counselling. In some cases, an antidepressant medication may help.

COUNSELLING

helps you to see problems in a new light, so that you can understand your emotions better. Counsellors offer a listening ear, helping you to explore your options and reach your own solutions – they don't usually advise you what to do or try to change you as a person. Counselling may help if your stress is related to:

- a specific short-term problem, such as a bereavement or a relationship breakdown
- a tangled web of emotions surrounding a particular situation
- a single, identifiable crisis.

PSYCHOTHERAPY

involves a more in-depth, longer course of treatment than counselling. It may explore what happened to you in the past and probe your subconscious feelings, memories, fears and fantasies. Techniques used include free association (reporting everything that comes into your head), transference (in which you 'transfer' emotions for other people onto the therapist to reveal subconscious anger, hurt or resentment) or hypnotherapy. Psychotherapy may help if your stress is associated with:

- deep dissatisfaction
- a long-standing problem
- lack of confidence
- you feeling cut off from your emotions
- a need to know yourself better.

COGNITIVE BEHAVIOUR THERAPY (CBT) is a form of psychotherapy that looks at how you think about yourself and other people, and how you respond to those thoughts and feelings. It helps you replace negative thought patterns and behaviours with more desirable ones. It focuses on the 'here and now' and how you currently feel, rather than on the past. CBT may be helpful if your stress is linked to:

- low self-esteem
- troublesome habits
- anger issues
- a social phobia
- panic attacks.

Here's an example of how CBT works. Your neighbour walks past while you're in the garden, and appears to ignore you. Having low self-esteem, you instantly think, 'She doesn't like me.' You go out of your way to stay indoors at the weekend, rather than sitting in the garden, listening to what sounds like a great party next door. Your self-esteem is now even lower than before.

CBT shows you more helpful ways to analyse the situation: perhaps your neighbour didn't say hello because her mind was on something else. Having good self-esteem, you feel concern for her (rather than for yourself). As a result, you pop round to check she's OK. In fact, she was distracted by plans for an impromptu barbecue, and instantly invites you to come and join them at the weekend.

'Wow, now that's what I call self-help!
Has it helped your wife's depression, too?'

DEALING WITH STRESS The ability to cope with stress isn't a trait that some lucky people have while others don't. It's a skill and, like any other skill, it improves with practice.

Here are the four main ways in which you can deal with excess pressure:

- remove or alter the source of stress
- change how you view the stressful event
- reduce the effects of stress on your body
- learn alternative ways to cope.

REMOVE OR ALTER THE SOURCE OF STRESS

A certain amount of stress keeps you on your toes, so aim to obtain the right balance between pressures you can handle and those you can't. Identify what causes you stress by keeping and analysing a stress diary. Examine each situation logically, put it into perspective and make sensible plans to resolve it. In most cases, this means learning people and time-management skills.

CHANGE HOW YOU VIEW THE STRESSFUL EVENT

Stress develops when the pressure you're under exceeds your comfort level. You can alter the balance by changing the way you perceive demands. If you believe you can deal with a stressful situation, you're likely to succeed. If you think you'll fail before you even begin, it becomes a self-fulfilling prophecy.

The trick is to view challenges as an opportunity, not as a threat. And if you do fail, welcome the opportunity to learn from your mistakes. It's all about taking control.

REDUCE THE EFFECTS OF STRESS

If you want to combat the effects of stress, it's vital to eat a healthy diet (see pages 24-25) to keep your body in good working order. So don't skip meals, no matter how busy you are.

Also find time to take regular exercise. Although a brisk walk may seem like a waste of time when you have deadlines looming, it will help to neutralize the effects of stress hormones. You'll feel refreshed and less tense, and will work more efficiently as a result. Double the benefit by using your walking time as thinking time.

Similarly, taking time out for relaxation is beneficial. These are all factors to be aware of:

- breathe slowly and calmly – watch out for hyperventilation
- explore the wide range of de-stressing complementary therapies (see pages 26-27 and 34-35)
- try not to rely on emotional crutches such as nicotine, alcohol or other recreational drugs.

LEARN ALTERNATIVE WAYS OF COPING

Several strategies can help you adapt to stress in a positive, constructive manner. Let go of unhelpful behaviours, such as avoidance. Putting your head in the sand, in the hope that things will go away, is counter-productive: anxiety usually builds up unless issues are properly resolved.

- Try not to blame everyone and everything else when things go wrong; projecting faults onto others means you lose the need to take responsibility and address the situation yourself.
- Accept valid criticism without taking it personally – use it as an opportunity to improve.
- Be aware and accept that it's OK to make mistakes; take responsibility and own up, give a personal commitment it won't happen again, and learn from the experience.
- Receive compliments with grace – don't downplay the positives (for example, by saying, 'I did that only through sheer luck').
- Avoid negative labels ('I'm a loser').
- Try not to jump to conclusions ('He must think I'm a loser').
- Change your use of language from 'I should do this ...', or 'I must do that ...' and 'I have to do the other ...' to 'I would like to do this today ...' or 'I would actually prefer to do that tomorrow'.

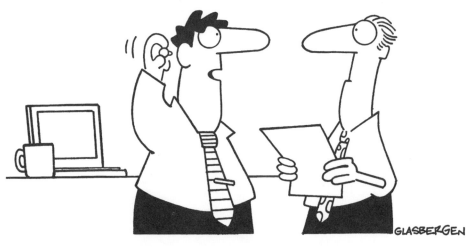

'It's a special hearing aid. It filters out criticism and amplifies compliments.'

21

MANAGING YOURSELF

Achieving balance is one of the cornerstones of stress reduction. If you're stressed and juggling too much, the amount of time you spend on the pleasurable things in life is almost certainly inadequate. Aim to spend less time in stress-causing situations and more time on exercise and relaxation – activities that reset your fight-or-flight reaction back to the rest-and-digest response. To do this, you need to manage yourself and your work/stress load.

When you feel in control, the pressure you experience is positive. But when the situation is in control of you, it leads to negative stress. Plan to take control. Make a 'To Do' list using a template such as those on pages 56–57. At the end of each day, plan your tasks for the next day in advance. This frees up the first part of your new day, when you are most fresh, for other tasks.

Most of us have too-busy lives. A 'To Do' list focuses your mind on outstanding tasks, allowing you to prioritize each activity and set a deadline for its completion. It also offers you the satisfaction of crossing out each task as it's completed. Add new tasks to the list as they arise. Then, at the end of each day, review your list and prioritize what you need to do the day after. Prioritizing tasks helps you to deal with pressures one at a time, starting with the most important, rather than drowning in an overwhelming sea of demands.

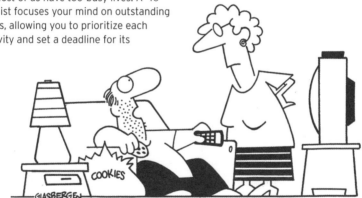

'I am not lazy! I am a potential workaholic
with highly developed stress-management skills!'

WORK TO LIVE, DON'T LIVE TO WORK

As you review your list, you'll notice tasks that keep recurring, or that tend to move up and down the list without getting crossed off when more important tasks take their place. Either DO them, REMOVE them or DELEGATE them. Don't keep putting them off – unfinished tasks contribute to your sense of time pressure.

DELEGATE! Delegation frees up your time and stress load by donating an activity to someone else who is equally capable – even if you think you can do it better yourself. For some people, delegation is easy, while others find it difficult to relinquish control. If you're one of the latter group, start practising.

ASSERT! Many stressed people find it difficult to say no. They take on too many tasks – perhaps from people who are themselves experts in delegation. Maintain control over your own obligations. Become comfortable with saying 'No', calmly and firmly, so that you don't take on more than you can cope with.

Being assertive without being aggressive is easy when you know how. Simply state your point pleasantly: 'I'm unable to work this weekend.' If the person reinforces their argument, do the same: 'I appreciate that's difficult for you, but I'm still unable to work this weekend.' Don't feel you have to apologize, or explain. Keep repeating yourself, like a cracked record. If you can, offer a compromise: 'I'm unable to work this weekend, but I'm happy to work next weekend if I can have time off in lieu.'

Recognize the difference between the things you MUST do, the things you SHOULD do and the things you NEED NOT do.

ANTI-STRESS DIET

Short-term stress mobilizes glucose and fatty acids in your body, so that you're ready for fighting or fleeing. In contrast, long-term stress drains you of energy, leaving you tired all the time. You may also eat erratically, skip meals and crave sweet, stodgy foods when under pressure.

GLYCAEMIC INDEX

The way different foods affect your blood glucose (sugar) levels is referred to as their glycaemic index (GI). Foods that rapidly increase blood glucose levels have a high GI, while foods that have a minimal impact on blood glucose levels have a low GI.

Eating foods with a high GI may seem a good idea if you are stressed and drained of energy, but it's not. A large rise in your glucose levels triggers release of insulin – a hormone that pushes glucose into the muscle and fat cells. When you produce too much insulin (which you tend to do on a high-GI diet), your blood glucose levels rebound too low, so you feel even more drained of energy.

Low glucose levels can produce sugar cravings, so you find yourself reaching for the biscuit tin. Unfortunately, eating more high-GI foods triggers the glucose-insulin cycle all over again. The stress hormone cortisol also reduces your response to insulin, so, in the long term, a rise in glucose levels increases your risk of type 2 diabetes.

START THE DAY RIGHT

Levels of the cortisol hormone are highest in the morning due to the physical 'stress' of your overnight fast. Eating a nutritious breakfast is therefore important to lower

---

ANTI-STRESS DIET TIPS

- Follow a low-GI diet
- Enjoy your food – eat slowly, sitting down
- Eat as wide a variety of foods as possible
- Eat the right amount to maintain a healthy weight
- Eat little and often – don't skip meals
- Eat at least five servings of fresh fruit and vegetables every day
- Cut back on sugar, salt and processed/convenience foods
- Concentrate on obtaining 'healthy' fats, such as olive oil, nut oils and rapeseed oil
- Eat at least two portions of oily fish per week
- Eat more beans and pulses

cortisol levels and set you up for the day. Yet many people skip breakfast, going without food for 15 hours or more. Surprisingly, they still expect their body and brain to function as normal.

For an ideal, anti-stress breakfast, select bran-based cereals, porridge, muesli, fruit, unsweetened yoghurt/fromage frais and skimmed or semi-skimmed milk.

Go easy on foods with a high GI and select foods with a low to moderate GI. Combine small amounts of food with a high GI (such as mashed potatoes) with those that have a lower GI (for example, beans) to help even out fluctuations in blood glucose levels.

FOOD WITH A HIGH GI – GO EASY

- Glucose
- Baked potatoes
- Potatoes, mashed
- White bread
- Parsnips
- Cornflakes
- Doughnuts
- Watermelon

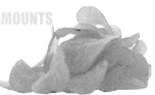

FOOD WITH A MEDIUM GI – EAT MODERATE AMOUNTS

- Basmati rice
- New potatoes, boiled
- Pineapple
- Honey
- Muesli
- Pitta bread
- Apricots
- Sultanas
- Potato crisps
- Porridge oats

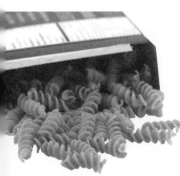

FOOD WITH A LOW GI – EAT FREELY

- Carrots
- Mangoes
- Bran cereal
- Green grapes
- Baked beans
- Oranges
- Pears
- Cherries
- Kiwi fruits
- Peas
- Milk
- Wholewheat pasta (cooked al dente)
- Apples

EXERCISING CONTROL
Exercise is one of the best ways to overcome anxiety and tension. It allows you to do exactly what the fight-or-flight response has prepared you for – physical exertion. This neutralizes the effects of stress hormones and helps switch you back into your rest-and-digest mode. Exercise also promotes relaxation by stimulating the release of opium-like endorphins in the brain.

Although exercise increases your blood pressure (BP) in the short term, in the long term it promotes the dilation of blood vessels. This reduces your blood pressure at rest and in situations that typically elevate BP such as emotional distress. It also has beneficial effects on cholesterol levels and glucose control. These effects soon wear off with inactivity, however, which is why regular exercise, preferably on a daily basis, is best.

YOGA
Yoga combines physical activity and relaxation to calm the body and relieve anxiety and stress. The stretching and relaxing of muscles it incorporates ease tension, while its breath-control techniques help to reduce the rapid breathing usually associated with hyperventilation and panic attacks (see pages 12-13).

Join a beginner's class, and gradually increase the number of sessions you attend (or perform at home) until you are practising yoga three or four times a week for at least 30 minutes per session. Adepts practise several times a day.

T'AI CHI
For something a bit different, try *t'ai chi*. This Chinese martial art involves slow, graceful movements, meditation and breathing techniques. As well as exercising the muscles, it promotes physical relaxation and emotional calm and has been described as meditation in motion. Research shows that *t'ai chi* can reduce stress and improve breathing efficiency.

As well as taking part in structured exercise, try to build more physical activity into your day: use the stairs rather than the lift or escalator; walk or cycle reasonable distances rather than taking the car; walk around the block in your lunch hour. If you can't get out and about, walk up and down the stairs or pace around your room several times a day.

If you have a strong drive to win, ensure any exercise you do is non-competitive or the stress of trying to win will counteract the benefits.

Don't overexercise, which can cause physical stress.

CHOOSE AN ACTIVITY TO SUIT YOU

- Walking – especially brisk walking or hillwalking
- Cycling
- Swimming
- Gym workout
- Jogging
- Gardening
- Golf
- Bowling
- Table tennis

- Dance class
- Keep-fit class
- Tennis
- Badminton
- Rambling
- A team sport such as netball, volleyball, football, rounders or baseball, cricket or hockey

When feeling particularly stressed, try the yoga posture known as *Savasana*.

- Lie down in a quiet, darkened room, on a carpeted floor or exercise mat, with your feet slightly apart.
- Let your arms lie comfortably by your sides, palms facing upwards.
- Breathe slowly and deeply, in and out through your nose, and feel a sense of calm wash through your whole body.

LIVING HEALTHILY

When you drive yourself hard to tick all the boxes and keep up with life's demands, it's easy to rely on quick fixes to chill you out. Alcohol and nicotine are common emotional crutches as, in small amounts, they have an initial calming effect. You may also be drawn to caffeine for a quick stimulant boost when prolonged stress drains you of energy. These props are false friends, however.

ALCOHOL Small amounts of alcohol can reduce stress levels, lower the blood pressure and lift your mood, but when you're stressed, your reliance on alcohol may increase. When your intake exceeds two or three units per day, your blood pressure increases, the pattern of sleep is adversely affected (so that you wake earlier, feeling less refreshed) and the harmful results of stress are magnified.

CAFFEINE Caffeine is a stimulant drug, the immediate effect of which is to reduce tiredness. This is thought to result from a direct action on the brain, which increases alertness and decreases the perception of effort and fatigue. However, caffeine also acts on the adrenal glands to increase circulating levels of the stress hormones adrenaline and cortisol. Excess caffeine makes you irritable, jittery and shaky. It also keeps you awake.

If you currently drink lots of caffeine-containing drinks, cut back gradually, over the course of a week. That will help you to avoid withdrawal symptoms such as restlessness, irritability, insomnia and headache.

SMALL AMOUNTS OF ALCOHOL CAN LOWER STRESS LEVELS

Aim to drink no more than one or two units of alcohol per day, and have at least two alcohol-free days per week.

BEVERAGE	CAFFEINE CONTENT PER AVERAGE SERVING
White tea	15mg
Green tea	25mg
Cola	45mg
Black tea	50mg
Instant coffee	60mg
Brewed coffee	100mg or more
Caffeinated high-energy drinks	150–400mg (check labels)

NICOTINE If you smoke, stress increases your need for nicotine, so you smoke more and more cigarettes when you're in a stressed state. Acute nicotine deprivation, which occurs within just 30 minutes of finishing a smoke, provokes increased feelings of stress, anger and irritability that can be reversed only by nicotine – in other words, by having another one. It's therefore difficult to quit 'cold turkey' when you are under pressure, unless you use nicotine-replacement therapy. The quit rate among people using nicotine patches, sprays, gums or microtabs is at least double that of people going it alone.

Keep a Quit Chart (see page 58) and tick off every day you keep within your target.

Caution: Don't smoke while you're using nicotine-replacement therapy. It could trigger dangerous spasm of the blood vessels and may even lead to a heart attack.

Aim to have no more than one cup of caffeinated coffee per day, plus three mugs of not-too-strong tea (preferably green or white tea). Ideally, slowly switch to decaffeinated brands, or drink herbal teas such as antioxidant-rich rooibos, calming camomile or soothing mint.

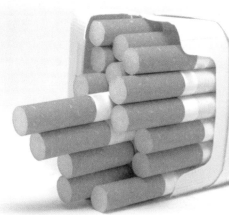

STRESS INCREASES NICOTINE CRAVINGS

BREATHING A SIGH OF RELIEF

The way you breathe is affected by stress hormones as part of the fight-or-flight response. When you experience prolonged stress, you tend to sigh deeply, gasp, hold your breath or breathe rapidly and shallowly.

If you persistently hyperventilate, this can lead to changes in blood acidity, which may trigger a panic attack (see pages 12–13). By learning to breathe properly instead, you can relieve some of the effects of stress, reduce your anxiety and achieve a more relaxed, tranquil approach to life.

Ask a friend to count your breathing rate when you are sitting down quietly, unaware. The average breathing rate is 10-12 breaths per minute. When hyperventilating you may breathe 15-20 times per minute, while someone who is panicking may take 30 breaths per minute or more. If you breathe 15 or more times per minute when at rest, consciously try to slow your breathing rate.

BREATH-AWARENESS EXERCISE

When you are stressed, you tend to breathe shallowly, using movements that involve only the upper part of your ribcage. Your shoulders tend to rise up towards your ears, with little expansion of your abdomen. You are also likely to hold your breath after inhaling and exhaling.

Whenever you begin to feel stress taking over, concentrate on breathing slowly and deeply, without holding your breath. And whenever you feel light-headed or panicky from a bout of overbreathing, cup your hands over your nose and mouth so that you can breathe back some of the excess carbon dioxide gas that you have exhaled. This will calmly and efficiently help to reduce any sense of panic.

To improve on your usual breathing technique:
- breathe into your diaphragm (so-called 'belly' breathing), rather than using shallow 'chest' breathing
- inhale through your nose
- exhale through your mouth
- take longer to exhale than to inhale
- don't hold your breath between inhaling and exhaling
- slow your breathing down so you take fewer breaths per minute
- practise over and over until this method of breathing becomes your natural pattern.

The following exercise will help you to achieve this:

- sit back comfortably in a chair and let your shoulders drop
- place one hand on your abdomen, and one hand on your upper chest
- as you breathe in and out, check that your lower hand rises first
- concentrate on the rise and fall of your abdomen rather than your chest
- now breathe in slowly and deeply; when you have inhaled fully, start to exhale immediately, without having held your breath; when you reach your limit of exhalation, start to breathe in again without holding your breath.
- breathing out should always take longer than breathing in. Get your rhythm right by slowly counting up to three when breathing in and slowly counting to four when breathing out.

Repeat this exercise, without holding your breath in-between, until you are confident that you recognize the difference between deep, even 'belly' breathing, and shallow, more stressed, chest breathing.

LEARN TO BREATHE PROPERLY AND YOU'LL ACHIEVE A MORE TRANQUIL APPROACH TO LIFE

TAKING IT EASY

When you're stressed, relaxation techniques can help you find inner calm. But relaxing is easier said than done. The pace of modern life means it's easy to lose the knack of switching off, without even realizing that it's gone.

CREATING PROMPTS

To signal the end of the working day and the beginning of 'me-time', create prompts that help you relax more quickly. Prepare your 'To Do' list for tomorrow, deciding what you need to prioritize and work on first. Tidy your work area (whether it's in an office or in the home) and think back on all that you've achieved today. Psychologically, this helps you feel the day is over.

Then, switch off for half an hour by reading, listening to soothing music or a talking book. This underlines that you've truly left your work behind. Rather than reaching for alcohol, have a relaxing herbal tea - camomile, mint, vanilla or rooibos are all ideal. You may also find it helpful to have a shower or aromatherapy bath (see page 34) before changing into

'something more comfortable'. It may be a bit of a cliché, but it really helps to get out of your work clothes as well as your work environment.

Try tuning in to your inner 'sound of silence', which resembles a high-pitched, constant tone. Once you are aware of it, and know how to find it, you can access it at any time (even in noisy surroundings) to help you relax when feeling stressed.

MINDFULNESS OF DECLUTTERING

Cleaning your house can reduce stress as you let go of things you no longer need. Approach decluttering as an exercise in mindfulness, rather than as a chore.

As you clear an area (on your desk or in your home), focus on what you're doing, as you're doing it, and think about nothing else. Feel the weight and texture of the objects in your hand; focus on the intensity of their colour; listen to the crackle of newspaper as you wrap delicate items; smell the scent of cardboard and enjoy the freedom of letting go as you place items in a box for charity.

CREATING A SANCTUARY Your home is your sanctuary, and creating a simple, uncluttered environment encourages calmness and tranquillity. Replicate nature's restful palate of greens, creams, beige, terracotta and cinnamon. Natural textures, such as linen, rattan, wood, stone and foliage, complete the relaxing air, while the presence of indoor plants has a positive effect on well-being and reduces feelings of stress. Create a peaceful atmosphere with flickering candles and CDs of natural sounds – lapping waves, babbling brooks, birdsong or tropical rain. And scent the air with relaxing aromatherapy essential oils (see pages 34-35).

MEDITATION Since ancient times, meditation has been used to reduce stress. It lowers the blood pressure and pulse rate and reduces stress hormones, while improving mood and anxiety. It allows you to focus on 'right now' rather than the future or the past.

But not everyone has time to sit with their eyes closed, quieting that little voice in their head. This is where mindfulness meditation comes in. It allows you to continue an activity while paying close attention to all the sensations, textures, colours, smells and sounds involved. This prevents your mind spinning off and dwelling on negative thoughts.

Another approach is to perform a task, such as decluttering (see opposite), while listening to relaxing music – whether you prefer orchestral, choral or 'chill-out' themes.

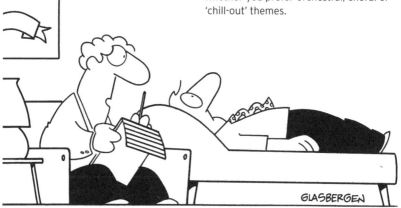

GLASBERGEN

'Meditation can bring you peace and serenity.
It gives you an excuse to look busy doing nothing.'

A LITTLE THERAPY GOES A LONG WAY
Many complementary therapies can reduce stress. Some techniques can be used for self-help, while others mean consulting a practitioner.

AROMATHERAPY uses essential oils, the intense aromas of which interact with your limbic system – a part of the brain involved in emotional responses. Anti-stress oils include basil, benzoin, bergamot, camomile, cedarwood, clary-sage, jasmine, lavender, marjoram, neroli, patchouli, rose, sandalwood, vanilla, vetiver and ylang-ylang.

Caution: Always dilute oils before use. Do not use essential oils if you are pregnant, except under specialist advice.

REFLEXOLOGY involves the massage of specific areas (called the reflexes) on the feet and hands. As well as being relaxing, it helps to relieve some stress-related problems such as headache, hyperventilation, digestive symptoms and panic attacks.

Add five drops of an essential oil blend to a tablespoon of carrier oil (for example, almond or avocado). Run a bath that is comfortably hot, then add the aromatic oil mix after turning off the taps. Soak for 15-20 minutes, preferably in candlelight.

WHEN SELECTING A COMPLEMENTARY PRACTITIONER

- Check that the practitioner is registered with the relevant umbrella organization. This ensures they have appropriate training, follow a code of ethics and have professional indemnity insurance.
- Find out how long your course of treatment will last and how much it will cost.

ACUPUNCTURE is based on the belief that life energy (*Qi*) flows through the body along channels known as meridians. Practitioners insert fine, disposable, sterile needles into acupoints overlying these meridians to regulate the flow of *Qi*. Acupuncture stimulates the release of endorphins – brain chemicals that reduce pain perception and stress. It is used to relieve stress-associated conditions such as headache, hyperventilation, anxiety, insomnia and addictions.

ACUPRESSURE is similar to acupuncture but involves massaging acupoints rather than stimulating them with needles.

THERAPEUTIC MASSAGE involves deep manipulation of body tissues to relieve tension, anxiety, high blood pressure, insomnia, low mood and other stress-related symptoms.

FLOWER REMEDIES use ultradilute flower essences preserved in grape alcohol (brandy) and can be taken to overcome stress and panic.

When you feel stressed, add five drops of your chosen flower essence to a glass of water and sip slowly, every three to five minutes, holding the liquid in your mouth for a while. Alternatively, place five drops directly on your tongue.

TO RELIEVE A TENSION HEADACHE WITH ACUPRESSURE

- Identify a point midway between your eyebrows, in the indentation between the bridge of your nose and forehead.
- Apply gentle steady pressure on this point, using your middle finger, making small rotations both clockwise and anticlockwise.
- Release the pressure after one minute, let your face muscles relax, and repeat once or twice more until the headache lifts.

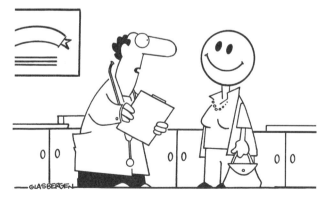

'St John's Wort is a great herb for improving your mood. But maybe it's time to cut back the dosage.'

ANTI-STRESS SUPPLEMENTS

The metabolic reactions associated with the fight-or-flight response quickly deplete the body of important vitamins and minerals, including vitamin C, the vitamin B group, calcium and magnesium. When under stress, a multivitamin and mineral supplement is a good idea as a nutritional safety net. Other nutritional supplements can also help.

SUPPLEMENT	BENEFIT	DAILY DOSE
B-group vitamins	Lack of B-group vitamins can lead to anxiety, irritability and fatigue and can make symptoms of stress worse. People with low levels of vitamin B_1 are also less likely to feel composed or self-confident and more likely to have low mood than those with higher levels.	25-50mg vitamin B complex
Vitamin C	Depletion of vitamin C contributes to reduced immunity and increased susceptibility to colds and other infections when you are stressed. Because vitamin C suppresses the activation of viral genes, viruses cannot survive in cells containing high levels of vitamin C. It also has an antioxidant action that reduces inflammation and hastens the healing process.	250mg-1g
Calcium	Low intakes of calcium are linked with sodium retention and high blood pressure. Alterations in calcium balance are associated with mood disturbances and clinical symptoms similar to those of premenstrual syndrome. Calcium may reduce some of the effects of stress through effects on brain neurotransmitters, including serotonin.	100-800mg

Magnesium	Depletion of magnesium may contribute to the fatigue and raised blood pressure associated with prolonged stress.	150–300mg
Probiotics	'Probiotics' is a term that describes the use of live 'friendly' organisms to confer a health benefit on the host. The most commonly used probiotics are lactic acid bacteria (LAB), such as certain strains of *Lactobacilli* and *Bifidobacteria*. These replenish immune-boosting bacteria in the gut and can reduce your chance of developing a cold during times of stress, when resistance is low. Taking probiotics plus a multivitamin and mineral significantly reduces the incidence and duration of cold and flu episodes.	One probiotic drink, which typically contains 1–5 billion colony-forming units (CFU) OR One enteric-coated supplement, which typically contains less (eg, 10 million freeze-dried probiotic bacteria)
Omega-3 fish oils	The omega-3 fatty acids DHA and EPA play an important role in brain function and mood regulation. Eating fish regularly can lift a low mood and neutralize some of the effects of excess stress by lowering stress hormone levels.	1–4g
5-HTP	5-HTP is converted into the 'happy' brain chemical, serotonin (5-HT), which helps to regulate mood, behaviour, appetite, sleep and impulse control. It helps to raise a low mood, reduce anxiety, improve sleep and relieve tension headache, and may also reduce the urge to 'comfort eat'.	50mg three times a day. After two weeks, increase to 100mg three times a day, if necessary For insomnia: 100–200mg before bedtime
Coenzyme Q10	CoQ10 is needed to process oxygen in cells, and to generate energy-rich molecules. It can improve physical energy and endurance, as well as helping to reduce blood pressure.	60–200mg

ANTI-STRESS SUPPLEMENTS

Many prescribed medicines are derived from plants. It is therefore not surprising that several herbal remedies are effective in relieving stress, promoting relaxation or providing a gentle stimulant effect.

HERB	BENEFIT	DAILY DOSE
Valerian	Valerian helps to relieve anxiety and muscle tension and promotes tranquillity. It is often combined with lemon balm to ease nervous anxiety, insomnia and reduce panic attacks.	250-800mg, two or three times a day (standardized to contain at least 0.8% valeric acid)
Camomile	Camomile has a soothing, relaxing action that reduces anxiety and promotes sleep.	1-3 cups of camomile tea
Lemon balm	Lemon balm is soothing and calming. It is traditionally used to reduce exam-related stress in students. It increases levels of an inhibitory brain chemical, GABA, that damps down anxiety.	650mg, three times a day
Oatstraw	Oatstraw is used as a restorative nerve tonic to help treat nervous exhaustion and stress. It is also used to reduce cravings in those who are quitting smoking.	1 dropper-full of fluid extract or tincture, two or three times a day
St John's Wort	St John's Wort helps to lift a low mood and may prove helpful where anxiety is associated with depression.	900mg (standardized to contain at least 0.3% hypericin or 3% hyperforin)
Guarana	Guarana contains a complex of natural stimulants, including caffeine. It increases energy levels and improves stress responses – usually without the jitteriness associated with other caffeine sources.	1g

ADAPTOGENS Many herbs are classed as 'adaptogens', meaning they help the adrenal gland to function and assist the body as it adapts to the effects of stress.

Ashwagandha	Ashwagandha is referred to as Indian ginseng. It is used in Ayurvedic medicine to improve resistance to stress. It also promotes serenity and deep sleep, especially in those suffering from overwork or nervous exhaustion.	150-300mg (standardized to contain 2-5mg of withanolides)
Astragalus	Astragalus is used in Chinese medicine to improve physical endurance and enhance immunity during times of stress.	250-500mg
Korean ginseng	Ginseng is stimulating and restorative, improving physical and mental energy, stamina, strength and alertness. Ginseng combines well with Ginkgo biloba to improve the memory and concentration.	200-600mg (in the East, ginseng is traditionally taken in a two weeks on/ two weeks off cycle
Reishi	Known as the mushroom of immortality, Reishi boosts physical and mental energy levels, lowers blood pressure, boosts immunity and promotes restful sleep.	500mg two or three times a day
Rhodiola	*Rhodiola* reduces anxiety and stress. It also has an energizing action to overcome stress-related fatigue and exhaustion.	400mg, once or twice a day
Siberian ginseng	Siberian ginseng works in similar ways to Korean ginseng. It acts as a restorative to enhance mental and physical function when tired and exhausted. It also boosts immunity against viral infections.	1-3g
Yerba maté	Yerba maté is used to overcome physical exhaustion and mental fatigue. It calms anxiety while improving concentration.	2-3 cups yerba maté tea daily

Caution: If you are taking any prescribed medicines, always check with a pharmacist or doctor before taking a herbal medicine, as interactions can occur.

LOWER YOUR

By reducing your stress levels, you will improve your quality and – most likely – your quantity of life. Following the 12-week stress-reduction programme is the first step towards becoming a new relaxed you.

WHY?

Stress increases your risk of developing a number of serious health problems. It also affects your physical, mental and social performance. If you recognize that you are stressed and don't do anything about it, you are heading towards total burn-out.

WHERE ARE YOU NOW?

In order to monitor your progress, it helps to assess your current status. So, before starting the 12-week stress-reduction programme, turn to pages 14–15. Count up all the early-warning signs and the psychological, emotional and physical symptoms that apply to you. Write the total in the Weekly Stress Symptoms Score Chart on page 58.

You should also make a mental note of any of the behavioural symptoms of stress that you recognize in yourself. You don't need to write them all down, but you can track your smoking, alcohol and caffeine habits using the charts on pages 58–59.

WHERE DO YOU WANT TO BE?

As you progress through your 12-week programme, you will become less and less stressed, and will feel considerably better than you do today. To keep track of your improvements, keep coming back and assessing your stress-related symptoms at the end of each week. Record these results in your Weekly Stress Symptoms Score Chart (see page 58).

You should notice a significant improvement as you reduce your stress load. This progress is entirely down to you – nobody else. Chalk this up as another achievement of which you can feel justly proud.

HOW ARE YOU GOING TO GET THERE?

Like all habits, continual negative thought patterns and harmful coping mechanisms are not easy to change. And, as discussed on pages 8–9, change is, in itself, a potent cause of stress.

It's therefore important that you don't try to alter too many of your familiar (yet

STRESS

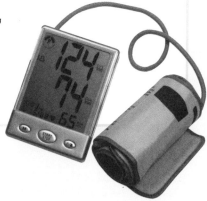

BEFORE STARTING THE PROCESS,

buy or borrow a home blood pressure-monitoring kit so you can keep an eye on your blood pressure. Record your blood pressure at the end of each day. If it is consistently above 140/90mmHg, see your doctor.

bad) habits too quickly. To accomplish changes in the long term and with the minimum amount of stress, it's best to tackle things slowly.

The Japanese have a useful philosophy, *kaizen*. It means committing yourself to making continuous, small steps towards improvement and is the ideal approach to take if you wish to reduce your stress levels.

Every week, your goal is to focus on a relatively easy technique that will help to reduce stress in your life. Each week also includes a lifestyle and therapy plan that will allow you to address some common causes of stress.

The good news is that after achieving each weekly stress-reducing goal you get to choose a reward to aid your motivation, such as a new book, DVD or CD, a manicure or facial, or a new DIY tool. Write your chosen reward in the allotted space for each week.

As you introduce each new change, you make sure you maintain the old changes so that, by the end of the programme, these new beneficial habits have become second nature.

The changes you made in the first few weeks will be more deeply ingrained than those you've made in the past few weeks. However, as you move forward in life, you will soon find that you do them all without thinking, reaping the benefits as you do so.

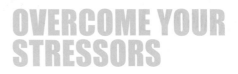

OVERCOME YOUR STRESSORS

Copy the Stress Diary Chart on pages 54-55, and fill it in every day this week (include changes in your blood pressure). Be honest and record events as objectively as possible (see pages 16-17). Keeping a stress diary helps to pinpoint the people or situations you find most stressful. It also provides insight into how you react to stress, so you can replace unhelpful coping patterns with more effective strategies. At the end of the week, review your stress diary and formulate plans to overcome each stressor in a positive way.

✓ LIFESTYLE TIP Now is the time to commit to taking regular brisk exercise – aim to fit at least 30 minutes into your day, every day (see pages 26-27). An energetic walk is an effective stress buster and can double up as useful thinking and planning time. If you're a smoker, also record the number of cigarettes you smoke each day in the chart on page 58. Try to cut back if you can, but it's more important to choose the right time to stop, which is why we address quitting properly when you are feeling less stressed, during Week 9.

◉ THERAPY Copy the weekly and daily 'To Do' charts from pages 56-57. List all the tasks you would like to complete this week in the weekly chart (see also pages 22-23). Then give each task a priority code: for example, 1 = urgent, 2 = soon, 3 = desirable but can wait. As new tasks come up, add them to your weekly list and code them accordingly. At the end of each day, prepare your 'To Do' tasks for tomorrow; plan to tackle the most urgent items first. Cross off each task as you complete it – it feels good.

Tick the chart on pages 60-61 for every day that you handle a stressful situation well.

🏆 **MY REWARD FOR THIS WEEK IS:** ....

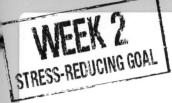

DELEGATE OR SHARE RESPONSIBILITIES

Hand over appropriate tasks to someone who is under less pressure than you are. You can still retain responsibility for the final result if you wish. But try not to add to your stress by micromanaging them as well as yourself. Share chores at home, using a rota if necessary. Consider investing in a cleaner, gardener or ironing service if these tasks are getting you down.

LIFESTYLE TIP Follow a healthy, low-glycaemic diet (see pages 24-25). Eat at least five servings of fruit and vegetables per day. Ensure you drink enough fluids, as dehydration reduces performance and can trigger tension headaches. An A-Z-style multivitamin and mineral supplement may help (see pages 36-37). Consider taking an adaptogen herb such as Siberian ginseng (see page 39).

THERAPY How often do you say 'Yes' and wish you hadn't? The easiest way to say 'No' is, in fact, not to use the word at all. Instead, say 'I am unable to ...' or 'I am unwilling to ...'.

Practise saying these phrases aloud until you feel comfortable. You are not rejecting the person, only their request. If it makes you feel better, say '... but thank you for asking' as you turn them down (see pages 22-23).

CONTINUE TO:
- Exercise every day
- Keep your weekly and daily 'To Do' list

Tick the chart on pages 60-61 for every day that you successfully say 'No' rather than 'Yes'.

🏆 MY REWARD FOR THIS WEEK IS: ....

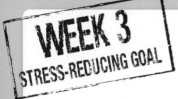

BE AWARE OF YOUR BREATHING

First, perform the breathing exercises on pages 30-31. Then, whenever you feel stressed, consciously slow your breathing rate down. This helps you feel more calm and relaxed.

✓ LIFESTYLE TIP Pay attention to your health. Make an appointment to see your doctor for a check-up. This will usually include blood pressure and cholesterol checks and a urine screen. If you think you may grind your teeth, have a dental check, too (see pages 14-15). And if you sit in front of a computer screen most days, visit an optometrist for an eye check.

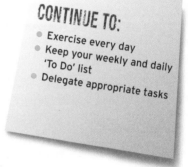

CONTINUE TO:
- Exercise every day
- Keep your weekly and daily 'To Do' list
- Delegate appropriate tasks

◉ THERAPY Work on improving your self-esteem. The most common negative self-belief is: 'I am not good enough.' Try not to compare yourself unfavourably with others. Instead, whenever you find yourself thinking, 'I can't do that', turn it round and say, 'I can do this.' Transform your negative thoughts into positive ones and you'll soon start believing in yourself. You *are* good enough.

Tick the chart on pages 60-61 for every day that you consciously check your breathing.

🏆 **MY REWARD FOR THIS WEEK IS:** ....

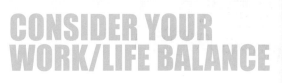

WEEK 4
STRESS-REDUCING GOAL

CONSIDER YOUR WORK/LIFE BALANCE

Plan to spend more time with those you love, doing things you enjoy. Designate at least one evening a week as 'Me Time' to do exactly what you like, when you like – whether it's meeting friends, reading a book or watching a good film. If necessary, organize a babysitter to cover for you. And build regular breaks into your day. You are more efficient when refreshed.

LIFESTYLE TIP Note how many caffeinated drinks you consume this week, using the chart on page 59. If you consume more than 300mg per day (see pages 28-29), you may have a caffeine addiction – cut back slowly to avoid stressful withdrawal. Make your drinks less strong by brewing them for a shorter length of time or adding fewer granules/tea leaves. Consider switching to decaffeinated brands. If you need a gentle caffeine boost, try guarana (see pages 38-39).

THERAPY Discuss emotions rather than bottling them up. Let family, friends and work colleagues know how you feel. When dealing with something that upsets you, use this simple formula: state what the problem is ('You didn't do X this morning'); state how this affects you ('I was late for work as I had to do X for you'); state how this makes you feel ('I feel annoyed and upset'); and state how you would like the issue resolved ('Please do X yourself in future').

CONTINUE TO:
- Exercise every day
- Keep your weekly and daily 'To Do' list
- Delegate appropriate tasks
- Be aware of your breathing

Tick the chart on pages 60-61 for every day that you spend more time on yourself.

🏆 **MY REWARD FOR THIS WEEK IS:** ....

CONSCIOUSLY RELAX

When feeling stressed, sit back comfortably in your chair or lie down. Close your eyes and breathe calmly and slowly. Let your attention roam over your body, consciously relaxing all of the muscles in your neck, hands, arms, shoulders, back, abdomen, bottom and legs. Sit or lie limply until you feel ready to face the world again.

✔ **LIFESTYLE TIP** Note how much alcohol you drink this week, filling in the chart on page 59. If you drink more than two units per day, plan to cut back. A good ploy is to avoid alcohol during the week or at least for a few days – say from Monday to Wednesday – and just have one or two drinks per day at weekends.

◉ **THERAPY** Anger can be appropriate, but try not to continue it beyond its natural expression. Allowing someone or something to make you angry means you lose control of your own emotions. Take responsibility for your own anger – you are in control of it, nobody else. Accept that you are angry, talk it out, then let it go. If you are too angry to think straight, move away from the situation temporarily. Say, 'I'll discuss this later', then take a brisk walk until your stress diffuses.

CONTINUE TO:
- Exercise every day
- Keep your weekly and daily 'To Do' list
- Delegate appropriate tasks
- Be aware of your breathing
- Look at your work/life balance

Tick the chart on pages 60-61 for every day that you consciously relax.

🏆 **MY REWARD FOR THIS WEEK IS:** ....

USE BIOFEEDBACK TO UNWIND

Take your resting pulse rate and blood pressure using your home BP monitor (see page 41). Now close your eyes and focus on bringing down your pulse rate. Visualize your heart beating in your chest and send it mental signals to go slow. After 10-15 minutes, take your pulse rate and BP again. A biofeedback device, such as the emWave Personal Stress Reliever (see Useful Websites on page 62), makes this easier by training you to synchronize your breathing and heart rate.

LIFESTYLE TIP Increase your level of exercise to at least 60 minutes per day (for example, 30 minutes' brisk walking plus 30 minutes' yoga, swimming or dancing). Consider cycling to work, the shops, meetings and friends' houses instead of taking the car – it's both good for the environment and good for you (see pages 26-27).

THERAPY When someone does something that irritates you, deal with it calmly and firmly before you get stressed. For example: 'John, I know you don't realize you're doing it, but please stop clicking that pen. It makes it hard for me to think straight. Could you put it down? Thanks.'

CONTINUE TO:
- Exercise every day
- Keep a weekly and daily 'To Do' list
- Delegate appropriate tasks
- Be aware of your breathing
- Look at your work/life balance
- Consciously relax (using biofeedback if you wish)

Tick the chart on pages 60-61 for every day that you take 60 minutes' exercise.

MY REWARD FOR THIS WEEK IS: ....

LEARN TO MEDITATE

Sit comfortably with your eyes closed. Visualize a colour such as white or purple. Focus on the colour, and try to clear your mind of intrusive thoughts. This becomes easier with practice. If your mind wanders, just return to focus on your chosen colour. When you feel ready, bring your mind slowly back. Stretch and enjoy the sense of calm energy and refreshment that flows through you. Try to meditate for at least 15 minutes a day. Or try mindfulness meditation as you go about your tasks (see pages 32-33).

✔ **LIFESTYLE TIP** Sprinkle a few drops of lavender essential oil on a tissue and inhale to promote sleep. A blend of lemongrass and neroli is also relaxing.

◉ **THERAPY** Accept constructive criticism. For example, 'Yes, I am sometimes late but I'm trying to be more punctual.' If the case against you is overstated ('You're always late'), calmly defend yourself: 'No, I'm not always late. I've been late only twice over the past few months.' Or ask for clarification: 'No, I am not always late. Why do you say that?' You will feel less stressed if you address the criticism appropriately.

CONTINUE TO:
- Exercise every day
- Keep a weekly and daily 'To Do' list
- Delegate appropriate tasks
- Be aware of your breathing
- Look at your work/life balance
- Consciously relax (using biofeedback if you wish)
- Monitor your blood pressure

Tick the chart on pages 60-61 for every day that you meditate.

🏆 **MY REWARD FOR THIS WEEK IS:** ....

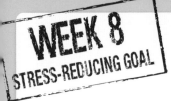
STOP WATCHING THE CLOCK

Avoid unnecessary time pressures by taking the clock off the wall and not wearing a watch. Experiment with missing a few of your less important deadlines – just to prove the world doesn't come to a grinding halt. In many cases, a deadline can be extended with little risk of disaster. Negotiate extensions to deadlines whenever you need more time to do the job properly.

✔ **LIFESTYLE TIP** Take time out to try a de-stressing complementary therapy – treat yourself to an aromatherapy massage, a reflexology treatment or an acupuncture session (see pages 34–35).

◉ **THERAPY** Bring more humour into your life. Laughter releases endorphins – the feel-good brain chemicals that can relieve stress and generally make you feel much happier and able to cope. Read a joke book, play light-hearted games with your family or friends or tune into a funny film or TV programme.

CONTINUE TO:
- Exercise every day
- Keep a weekly and daily 'To Do' list
- Delegate appropriate tasks
- Be aware of your breathing
- Look at your work/life balance
- Consciously relax (using biofeedback if you wish)
- Monitor your blood pressure
- Meditate regularly

Tick the chart on pages 60–61 for every day that you stop watching the clock.

🏆 **MY REWARD FOR THIS WEEK IS:** ....

FOCUS ON YOUR GOOD POINTS

Comparing yourself unfavourably to others is a powerful source of internal stress. Overcome this by writing down at least ten qualities you like about yourself: a good sense of humour, committed, caring, loyal, flexible, adaptable, intelligent ... The list could go on and on. No one can take these qualities away from you. Put the list in your wallet or purse and read it the next time you feel someone is better than you. Keep adding to the list as you discover more qualities that make you feel good about yourself.

✔ **LIFESTYLE TIP** If you smoke, do your utmost to quit now you've followed the programme for eight weeks and are less stressed. Those who make a Quit Plan are twice as likely to succeed as those who just stop without thinking things through properly. It helps to cut back on the number of cigarettes you smoke in the lead-up to your Quit Day. See pages 28–29, and use the Quit Smoking Chart on page 58.

◎ **THERAPY** Instead of looking for excuses to be disappointed, look for reasons to say 'Thank you' or 'Well done'. When you help others feel good about themselves, the effects rub off on you, too.

CONTINUE TO:
- Exercise every day
- Keep a weekly and daily 'To Do' list
- Delegate appropriate tasks
- Be aware of your breathing
- Look at your work/life balance
- Consciously relax (using biofeedback if you wish)
- Monitor your blood pressure
- Meditate regularly
- Negotiate longer deadlines

Tick the chart on pages 60–61 for every day that you focus on your good points.

🏆 **MY REWARD FOR THIS WEEK IS:** ....

REVIEW YOUR 'TO DO' LISTS

Are you prioritizing tasks appropriately? Are you doing, delegating or removing tasks that keep recurring, or which don't quite get done (see pages 22-23)? Are you shaping your own day rather than responding to other people's demands on your time? If you find yourself juggling several half-finished tasks, try doing only one thing at a time and completing it before moving on to the next.

✅ **LIFESTYLE TIP** Declutter your home and work environment. Keep your work surfaces clean and tidy. Do this mindfully (see pages 32-33). Handle papers as little as possible – file them as soon as you've read and assessed them; this saves dealing with them again later. Try surrounding yourself with green plants (again, see pages 32-33).

◉ **THERAPY** Try not to downplay your achievements – be comfortable accepting praise. Congratulate others on their success and allow yourself to feel happy for them. Their success does not detract from your own skills and abilities in any way.

CONTINUE TO:
- Exercise every day
- Keep a weekly and daily 'To Do' list
- Delegate appropriate tasks
- Be aware of your breathing
- Look at your work/life balance
- Consciously relax (using biofeedback if you wish)
- Monitor your blood pressure
- Meditate regularly
- Negotiate longer deadlines
- Focus on your good points

Tick the chart on pages 60-61 for every day that you prioritize tasks properly.

🏆 **MY REWARD FOR THIS WEEK IS:** ....

DON'T JUDGE YOURSELF TOO HARSHLY

Are you too much of a perfectionist? Sometimes, second best is more than good enough. If you believe your performance is poor, are you being too critical? Where is the evidence? Ask other people what they think, and use their feedback in a positive, constructive manner. Improve your performance where you can, otherwise accept that you did as well as you could, using the time and resources available.

LIFESTYLE Consider enrolling in an evening class to learn a new skill: acting, sculpture, painting, life drawing or even a yachting Day Skipper course. If you don't like your job, retrain for something else. Or use the time for more exercise by joining a yoga, *t'ai chi* or salsa dancing class. A new hobby helps you climb out of a stressful rut.

THERAPY Avoid using words that exaggerate events. Make molehills out of mountains, rather than the other way round. Instead of 'terrible', say 'inconvenient'; instead of 'dreadful', say 'annoying'; for 'awful', try 'unfortunate'; in place of 'I have to', use 'I would like to'; and instead of 'I must', say 'I intend to'.

CONTINUE TO:

- Exercise every day
- Keep a weekly and daily 'To Do' list
- Delegate appropriate tasks
- Be aware of your breathing
- Look at your work/life balance
- Consciously relax (using biofeedback if you wish)
- Monitor your blood pressure
- Meditate regularly
- Negotiate longer deadlines
- Focus on your good points
- Review your 'To Do' lists

Tick the chart on pages 60–61 for every day that you accept you are doing your best

🏆 MY REWARD FOR THIS WEEK IS: ....

ADDRESS CONTINUING STRESSORS

Keep a stress diary again this week. Copy the chart on pages 54–55 and fill it in every day (again, include changes in your blood pressure). Things should have noticeably changed for the better since the last time you did this during Week 1. Consider which people or situations are causing you the most stress now. Formulate new plans to overcome each stressor in a positive way.

LIFESTYLE TIP An ancient Chinese technique can help to relieve stress. Imagine something that makes you happy, and smile internally so it is felt only by you. It doesn't have to be visible. Let the smile shine out of your eyes and travel inwards to spread all over your body before concentrating the feeling just below your navel. As the smile radiates within, it generates a feeling of relaxation and peace.

THERAPY No one can make you feel inferior without you letting them – how you respond to negative remarks is up to you and you alone. Believe in yourself!

CONTINUE TO:

- Exercise every day
- Keep a weekly and daily 'To Do' list
- Delegate appropriate tasks
- Be aware of your breathing
- Look at your work/life balance
- Consciously relax (using biofeedback if you wish)
- Monitor your blood pressure
- Meditate regularly
- Negotiate longer deadlines
- Focus on your good points
- Review your 'To Do' lists
- Judge yourself more kindly and accept that you are doing your best

Tick the chart on pages 60–61 for every day that you manage your stressors appropriately.

MY REWARD FOR THIS WEEK IS: ....

STRESS DIARY CHART

Date: **Day:** Monday   Tuesday   Wednesday

Time of day	Intensity of stress (1-10)	Situation (causes, places, people)	How I felt

* If your blood pressure is consistently higher than 140/90mmHg, see your doctor to discuss whether or not you need treatment

Thursday	Friday	Saturday	Sunday

Negative responses (including rises in blood pressure*)

Possible solutions

'TO DO' CHARTS

Use whichever of these formats suit your purposes best – or design your own.

WEEKLY PLANNER   Week commencing

TO DO BY: **TASK:**   **NOTES:**

Monday

Tuesday

Wednesday

Thursday

Friday

Saturday

Sunday

DAILY 'TO DO' LIST You can use a similar format for your weekly 'To Do' list, too, if you prefer. Add tasks as they arise, and transfer the most important to a daily 'To Do' list at the end of each day, ready for tomorrow.

PRIORITY:
1, 2 or 3

DAILY 'TO DO' LIST

TASK:	PRIORITY: 1, 2 or 3	DONE ✓

HEALTH CHARTS

WEEKLY STRESS SYMPTOMS SCORE CHART Record the number of symptoms experienced at the start, before you begin the programme, and at the end of each week.

WEEK	START	1	2	3	4	5	6	7	8	9	10	11	12
Number of symptoms													

QUITTING SMOKING CHART Take it one day at a time. Record the number of cigarettes smoked each day, or tick off each cigarette-free day.

WEEK	Day 1	Day 2	Day 3	Day 4	Day 5	Day 6	Day 7
1							
2							
3							
4							
5							
6							
7							
8							
9							
10							
11							
12							

QUIT TIPS The physical cravings caused by nicotine usually disappear within seven days, but the psychological 'need' lasts longer. Expect the first three to four days to be the hardest. Those who make a Quit Plan are twice as likely to succeed as those who just stop without thinking things through properly. It helps if you try to cut back on the number of cigarettes you smoke in the lead up to Quit Day.

- Throw away all smoking-related items such as cigarettes, rolling papers, matches, lighters and ashtrays.
- Find support – it's easier to quit together with a friend or relative who also wants to give up.
- Keep your hands busy with a stress-relief ball, model-making, painting, origami, knitting or do-it-yourself repairs. These activities will help you to overcome the psychological hand-to-mouth habit that makes quitting so difficult.
- Think smart and avoid situations where you used to smoke.
- Learn to say, 'No thanks, I've given up' or 'No thanks, I'm cutting down.'
- When you feel the urge to smoke, eat an apple, clean your teeth and/or take some brisk exercise instead.

WEEKLY ALCOHOL CHART

DAY	Alcoholic drinks	Number of units*
Monday		
Tuesday		
Wednesday		
Thursday		
Friday		
Saturday		
Sunday		

*Calculate using the drinks tracker at www.drinkaware.co.uk

WEEKLY CAFFEINE CHART

DAY	Caffeinated drinks	Amount of caffeine (mg)*
Monday		
Tuesday		
Wednesday		
Thursday		
Friday		
Saturday		
Sunday		

*See caffeine content of drinks on page 29

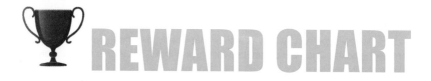

REWARD CHART

WEEK DAY/GOAL	1 HANDLE A STRESSFUL SITUATION WELL	2 SAY 'NO' RATHER THAN 'YES'	3 CHECK YOUR BREATHING	4 SPEND MORE TIME ON YOURSELF	5 RELAX	6 CONSCIOUSLY TAKE 60 MINUTES OF EXERCISE
Monday						
Tuesday						
Wednesday						
Thursday						
Friday						
Saturday						
Sunday						

WEEK COMPLETED REWARD STAR Colour in or stick on a gold star

MY CHOSEN REWARD FOR THIS WEEK IS:

For every day that you successfully complete that week's task, give yourself a tick in the following boxes. Once you complete a full week of ticks, you earn a gold star and can access the weekly reward you promised yourself.

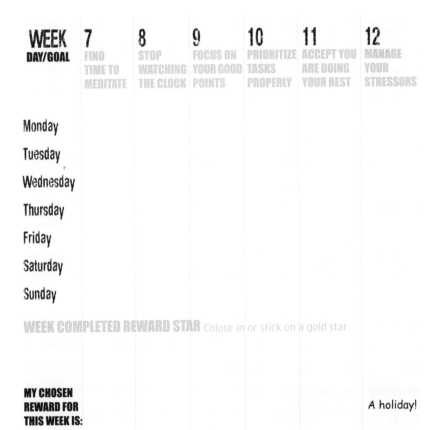

WEEK	7	8	9	10	11	12
DAY/GOAL	FIND TIME TO MEDITATE	STOP WATCHING THE CLOCK	FOCUS ON YOUR GOOD POINTS	PRIORITIZE TASKS PROPERLY	ACCEPT YOU ARE DOING YOUR BEST	MANAGE YOUR STRESSORS
Monday						
Tuesday						
Wednesday						
Thursday						
Friday						
Saturday						
Sunday						

WEEK COMPLETED REWARD STAR Colour in or stick on a gold star

| MY CHOSEN REWARD FOR THIS WEEK IS: | | | | | A holiday! | |

USEFUL WEBSITES

Visit www.naturalhealthguru.co.uk to read more health information from me, Dr Sarah Brewer. You can also email me via this site to let me know how well you've succeeded by following the Cut Your Stress programme. Follow my daily nutritional tweets at www.twitter.com/DrSarahB

STRESS

American Academy of Experts in Traumatic Stress www.aaets.org
American Institute of Stress www.stress.org
Anxiety UK www.anxietyuk.org.uk
British Association for Behavioural and Cognitive Psychotherapies www.babcp.com
British Association for Counselling and Psychotherapy www.bacp.co.uk
British Psychological Society www.bps.org.uk
International Stress Management Association (UK) www.isma.org.uk
National Association of Cognitive-Behavioral Therapists (US) www.nacbt.org
No Panic www.nopanic.org.uk
UK Council for Psychotherapy www.psychotherapy.org.uk

BIOFEEDBACK

emWave www.emWavepc.com; www.heartmathstore.com

BLOOD PRESSURE

American Society of Hypertension www.ash-us.org
Blood Pressure Association (UK) www.bpassoc.org.uk
European Society of Hypertension www.eshonline.org

SMOKING

Action on Smoking and Health UK www.ash.org.uk
Action on Smoking and Health US www.ash.org
Quit UK www.quit.org.uk

ALCOHOL

Alcohol Concern www.alcoholconcern.org.uk
Drink Aware Trust www.drinkaware.co.uk
National Institute on Alcohol Abuse and Alcoholism (US) www.niaaa.nih.gov

COMPLEMENTARY THERAPIES

Alternative Medicine Foundation (US) www.amfoundation.org
American Association of Integrative Medicine www.aaimedicine.com
British Complementary Therapies Council www.bctcvsr.org.uk
Complementary and Natural Healthcare Council (UK) www.cnhc.org.uk
Complementary Medical Association www.the-CMA.org.uk

INDEX

The information in this book is not a substitute for professional medical or health care. The advice in this book is based on the training, expertise and information available to the author. Each personal situation is unique. The author and publisher urge the readers to consult a qualified health professional when there is any question regarding the presence or treatment of any health condition. Unless otherwise specified the treatments recommended are for use by adults. Pregnant women should always consult a qualified health professional before using any treatments recommended in this publication.

The author and publisher are not responsible for any adverse effects or consequences resulting from the use of any of the preparations or procedures described in this book. For personalised advice, please always consult a qualified health professional. Research studies and institutions cited in this book should in no way be construed as an endorsement of anything in this book. The author and publisher expressly disclaim responsibility for any adverse effects arising from the use or application of the information contained herein.

Picture credits

Cartoons © Randy Glasbergen 5, 11, 12, 19, 21, 22, 33 and 35; iStockphoto/Ivan Montero 7, 23 (top), 25 and 35; iStockphoto 9; Science photo library/Victor De Schwanberg 12; Science photo library/James King-Holmes 15; iStockphoto/Paul Turner 18; iStockphoto/Stefanie Timmermann 19 (top); iStockphoto 19 (centre); iStockphoto/Jacob Wackerhausen 19 (bottom); iStockphoto 20; iStockphoto/Mark Jensen 23 (bottom); iStockphoto 24; Stockphoto 29; iStockphoto/Feng Yu 30; iStockphoto/Nicholas Monu 32; iStockphoto/Hermann Danzmayr 34; iStockphoto/Craig Veltri 41; iStockphoto 42-53

Quercus Editions Ltd
21 Bloomsbury Square
London WC1A 2NS

First Published 2010

Concept, text, design and layout © Quercus Editions Ltd 2010

The picture credits constitute an extension to this copyright notice.

A catalogue record for this book is available from the British Library.

ISBN: 978-1-84866-064-9

Printed in China

Every effort has been made to contact copyright holders. However, the publishers will be glad to rectify in future editions any inadvertent omissions brought to their attention.

Text by Dr Sarah Brewer
Edited by Ali Moore
Designed by Jane McKenna